Prayer

SUPERNATURAL
CHILDBIRTH

by

Jackie Mize

Harrison House
Tulsa, Oklahoma

Unless otherwise indicated all Scripture quotations are taken from the *King James Version* of the Bible.

17 16   17 16 15

Prayers and Promises for Supernatural Childbirth
ISBN-13: 978-1-57794-767-7
ISBN-10: 1-57794-767-3

Copyright © 2005 by Jackie Mize
P. O. Box 35044
Tulsa, OK 74153

Published by Harrison House Publishers
P. O. Box 35035
Tulsa, Oklahoma 74153

Preface

To Jackie and me the words "supernatural child-birth" aren't just a catchy phrase or a sermon title. These words to us mean Lynn, Paul, Lori, and Cristy. Supernatural childbirth to us means faith in God's Word to bring about what man has declared impossible.

When Jackie and I met and began talking marriage, she said to me, "If we are going to get married, there is something about me you should know."

"I CAN'T HAVE CHILDREN!" she said.

What a devastating statement! Women around the world have made the same declaration. My question to them now is the same question I posed to Jackie over two decades ago. "Oh, really? Who said? Who said you can't have children?" It makes a major difference in every area of your life, who said. I am always asking people that question, "Who said?"

Jackie answered me, "The doctors said."

"Oh, I see. Well, God said you can have babies," I told her. "Even though I thank God for doctors and hospitals, and medical science is always advancing, they are not our source, our final authority; God is, and God said you can have children."

"He did?"

"Sure. The Bible is full of Scriptures about children. He said He makes the barren woman to keep house and be a joyful mother of children. He said your children will be as olive plants and your wife as a fruitful vine. The Bible says there will be neither male nor female barren among God's people. We will have all the children we want."

And we did. We have four children—two boys and two girls. And we've taken them around the world with us giving Living Bread to dying men, sharing the gospel with the world that cost the blood of Jesus.

Jackie's testimony of supernatural childbirth has gone literally around the world. In many nations where I go, people come up to me and say, "I've heard your wife's tape on supernatural childbirth." We have files of testimonies from women at home and abroad who have beautiful children because they applied these faith principles from God's Word. We strongly believe that any man, woman, boy, or girl can take God's Word and change his/her circumstances through faith and prayer.

Something that Jackie and I want people to understand is that to us, supernatural childbirth is being able to believe God to get pregnant, carry that baby to full term, and have a healthy mommy deliver a healthy baby. Many people think that supernatural childbirth only means having painless childbirth because that is what Jackie did with three of our four children; but we've never been dogmatic about that. Our point is having the baby and being healthy. The painless part and all the other extras we've had and believed for are available for you as you use your faith and "shoot for the stars; go for the best; aim high!" Those are faith principles. With God and faith you can always go all out and aim high. The bottom line is this: the Bible says, "According to your faith." There isn't a right way and a wrong way in this book. There isn't "Jackie's way." It's according to your faith. We got what we used our faith for. We believe you will too!

—*Terry L. Mize*

Introduction

The Importance of Confession

Confesssion is an important act of faith on your part. There are over 3,000 Scriptures concerning words, mouth, tongue, lips, say, and speak. Surely God must be trying to tell us something.

Confession is not new; it's as old as the Bible. It's not strange, foreign, dark, or mysterious. Confession is simply agreeing out loud with God, saying what God has already said.

When we pray, we must pray the Word, and pray in agreement with God's Word. We have God's Word for every area of our life; now it's up to us to make our own words agree with God's written Word. Jesus prayed, "Not my will but Yours be done." Well, we have the will of God, the Bible. We know God's will;

now we must give voice to it in our prayers and in our everyday lives.

The Bible says:

Death and life are in the power of the tongue: and they that love it shall eat the fruit thereof.

Proverbs 18:21

Thou art snared with the words of thy mouth, thou art taken with the words of thy mouth.

Proverbs 6:2

And this is the confidence that we have in him, that, if we ask any thing according to his will, he heareth us:

And if we know that he hear us, whatsoever we ask, we know that we have the petitions that we desired of him.

1 John 5:14,15

I call heaven and earth to record this day against you, that I have set before you life and death, blessing and cursing: therefore choose life, that both thou and thy seed may live.

Deuteronomy 30:19

For verily I say unto you, That whosoever shall say unto this mountain, Be thou removed, and be thou cast into the sea; and shall not doubt in his heart, but shall believe that those things which he saith shall come to pass; he shall have whatsoever he saith.

Mark 11:23

Generation of vipers, how can ye, being evil, speak good things? for out of the abundance of the heart the mouth speaketh.

Matthew 12:34

Terry and I vowed to God long ago, "We will make our words agree with Your Word in every area—marriage, children, family, health, finances, ministry—and if we don't know what Your Word says on a given subject, we won't say anything until we look it up in the Bible, then we'll say what the Bible says!"

Here is what God has said about you and your baby. Now you agree with Him.

Listed below are some Scriptures and confessions we made daily during pregnancy and some others concerning our family and ministry that we still use, pray, confess, agree with, and declare, and have for over two decades. In fact, if you wanted a formula or recipe for our lives and ministry, you could blend these Scriptures and confessions together, add in the Great Commission, plus the previous Scriptures I've already given you, and you would get Terry and Jackie Mize, our life and ministry.

> This book of the law shall not depart out of thy mouth; but thou shalt meditate therein day and night, that thou mayest observe to do according to all that is written therein: for then thou shalt make thy way prosperous, and then thou shalt have good success.
>
> Joshua 1:8

> Then said the Lord unto me, Thou hast well seen: for I will hasten my word to perform it.
>
> Jeremiah 1:12

> I will worship toward thy holy temple, and praise thy name for thy lovingkindness and for thy truth: for thou hast magnified thy word above all thy name.
>
> Psalm 138:2

My son, attend to my words; incline thine ear unto my sayings. Let them not depart from thine eyes; keep them in the midst of thine heart.

For they are life unto those that find them, and health to all their flesh.

Proverbs 4:20-22

It is vital that you take the Word of God and declare it from your own mouth. There is no such thing as an unimportant word or a word void of power.

I can do all things through Christ which strengtheneth me.

Philippians 4:13

But my God shall supply all your need according to his riches in glory by Christ Jesus.

Philippians 4:19

For by him were all things created, that are in heaven, and that are in earth, visible and invisible, whether they be thrones, or dominions, or principalities, or powers: all things were created by him, and for him.

Colossians 1:16

The thief cometh not, but for to steal, and to kill, and to destroy: I am come that they might have life, and that they might have it more abundantly.

John 10:10

Thou art worthy, O Lord, to receive glory and honour and power: for thou hast created all things, and for thy pleasure they are and were created.

Revelation 4:11

Being confident of this very thing, that he which hath begun a good work in you will perform it until the day of Jesus Christ.

Philippians 1:6

Let us hold fast the profession of our faith without wavering; (for he is faithful that promised.)

Hebrews 10:23

Draw nigh to God, and he will draw nigh to you. Cleanse your hands, ye sinners; and purify your hearts, ye double-minded.

James 4:8

For with God nothing shall be impossible.

Luke 1:37

Blessed is the man that walketh not in the counsel of the ungodly, nor standeth in the way of sinners, nor sitteth in the seat of the scornful.

But his delight is in the law of the LORD; and in his law doth he meditate day and night.

And he shall be like a tree planted by the rivers of water, that bringeth forth his fruit in his season; his leaf also shall not wither; and whatsoever he doeth shall prosper.

Psalm 1:1-3

And Jesus answered him, saying, It is written, That man shall not live by bread alone, but by every word of God.

Luke 4:4

How God anointed Jesus of Nazareth with the Holy Ghost and with power: who went about doing good, and healing all that were oppressed of the devil; for God was with him.

Acts 10:38

For with the heart man believeth unto righteousness; and with the mouth confession is made unto salvation.

Romans 10:10

Nay, in all these things we are more than conquerors through him that loved us.

Romans 8:37

And be not conformed to this world: but be ye transformed by the renewing of your mind, that ye may prove what is that good, and acceptable, and perfect, will of God.

Romans 12:2

Who his own self bare our sins in his own body on the tree, that we, being dead to sins, should live unto righteousness: by whose stripes ye were healed.

1 Peter 2:24

Give, and it shall be given unto you; good measure, pressed down, and shaken together, and running over, shall men give into your bosom. For with the same measure that ye mete withal it shall be measured to you again.

Luke 6:38

Bring ye all the tithes into the storehouse, that there may be meat in mine house, and prove me now herewith, saith the Lord of hosts, if I will not open you the windows of heaven, and pour you out a blessing, that there shall not be room enough to receive it.

And I will rebuke the devourer for your sakes, and he shall not destroy the fruits of your ground; neither shall your vine cast her fruit before the time in the field, saith the Lord of hosts.

Malachi 3:10,11

Beloved, I wish above all things that thou mayest prosper and be in health, even as thy soul prospereth.

3 John 2

Surely he hath borne our griefs, and carried our sorrows: yet we did esteem him stricken, smitten of God, and afflicted.

But he was wounded for our transgressions, he was bruised for our iniquities: the chastisement of our peace was upon him; and with his stripes we are healed.

Isaiah 53:4,5

And all thy children shall be taught of the Lord; and great shall be the peace of thy children.

In righteousness shalt thou be established: thou shalt be far from oppression; for thou shalt not fear: and from terror; for it shall not come near thee.

Behold, they shall surely gather together, but not by me: whosoever shall gather together against thee shall fall for thy sake.

Isaiah 54:13-15

No weapon that is formed against thee shall prosper; and every tongue that shall rise against thee in judgment thou shalt condemn. This is the heritage of the servants of the Lord, and their righteousness is of me, saith the Lord.

Isaiah 54:17

Use the following verses from Galatians to negate the curses of the Law found especially in Deuteronomy chapter 28.

Christ hath redeemed us from the curse of the law, being made a curse for us: for it is written, Cursed is every one that hangeth on a tree:

That the blessing of Abraham might come on the Gentiles through Jesus Christ; that we might receive the promise of the Spirit through faith.

And if ye be Christ's, then are ye Abraham's seed, and heirs according to the promise.

Galatians 3:13,14,29

Now don't forget the Great Commission found in Matthew 28:19,20; Mark 16:15-18; Luke 24:47; John 20:21; and Acts 1:8.

Confessions
and
Prayers

Dealing With Fear
and Thoughts

Fear is a spiritual force. It is the opposite of faith. Fear is real, and it is not of God. It affects the life we live on planet earth. It affects the physical body. It can put a wrinkle in the skin, change the color of hair, make the heart beat fast or even stop. It has killed many people over the years. The Bible says in the last days men's hearts will fail them for fear. (Luke 21:26.) Fear motivates Satan as faith motivates God. Fear is Satan's tool as faith is God's.

You only fear the unknown or past bad experiences. Past failures bring future fears. Fear and faith don't operate together. Fear is your worst enemy when it's allowed to operate. It can be one of the greatest causes of pain during childbirth.

Now don't get scared. I've got good news for you. Actually, the Word of God has good news for you.

The Bible says in 1 John 4:18 that fear has torment but perfect love casts out fear. Now, God is love (1 John 4:16) the Bible says, and you've got God, so fear must go.

Second Timothy 1:7 says, "For God hath not given us the spirit of fear; but of power, and of love, and of a sound mind." You can conquer fear in Jesus' name with faith in God's Word. And Romans 10:17 says, "So then faith cometh by hearing, and hearing by the word of God."

All through the Bible God says, "Fear not...." "Don't be afraid...." Doesn't it make sense that when you are at peace, your body will be relaxed; it can stretch more, be more elastic? On the other hand, fear causes your body and muscles and nerves to tense up, to tighten. Jesus said, "My peace I leave with you." (John 14:27.) Faith in God's Word brings peace.

F—alse

E—vidence

A—bout

R—eality

Prayer/Confession

Father, I come before You in the mighty name of Jesus and the covenant of blood, and I rebuke fear and doubt and unbelief. Your Word says You have not given me a spirit of fear but of love and power and a sound mind. Your Word also says that fear has torment but that perfect love casts out fear and God is love; and I've got God living big in me so fear and torment go far from me now, in Jesus' name. I trust in the Lord; I will not fear; I will not be afraid. I have the mind of Christ and the peace of God. My mind and body, as well as my spirit, are relaxed and at peace. I refuse to let my heart be troubled or afraid.

The Lord, Most High, is my light and my salvation, whom shall I fear? The Lord, El Shaddai, is the strength of my life, of whom shall I be afraid?

Body, I speak to you to be at peace, relax, rest. Muscles, nerves, be at peace. I rest in faith in God's Word and thank You, Father, for total and complete peace and confidence, in Jesus' name. Amen. (Ps. 112:7; Isa. 41:10; Ps. 27:1; Isa. 54:17; John 14:27; 1 John 4:18; Phil. 4:7,8; Eph. 4:27; Isa. 26:3; 1 Peter 5:7.)

Here are some more Scriptures for you to think on and to confess.

When thou liest down, thou shalt not be afraid: yea, thou shalt lie down, and thy sleep shall be sweet.

Proverbs 3:24

I sought the LORD, and he heard me, and delivered me from all my fears.

Psalm 34:4

And to you who are troubled rest with us, when the Lord Jesus shall be revealed from heaven with his mighty angels.

2 Thessalonians 1:7

Casting down imaginations, and every high thing that exalteth itself against the knowledge of God, and bringing into captivity every thought to the obedience of Christ.

2 Corinthians 10:5

No weapon that is formed against thee shall prosper; and every tongue that shall rise against thee in judgment thou shalt condemn. This is the heritage of the servants of the Lord, and their right-eousness is of me, saith the Lord.

Isaiah 54:17

He sent his word, and healed them, and delivered them from their destructions.

Psalm 107:20

Let us therefore come boldly unto the throne of grace, that we may obtain mercy, and find grace to help in time of need.

Hebrews 4:16

And be not conformed to this world: but be ye transformed by the renewing of your mind, that ye may prove what is that good, and acceptable, and perfect, will of God.

Romans 12:2

For I know the thoughts that I think toward you, saith the Lord, thoughts of peace, and not of evil, to give you an expected end.

Jeremiah 29:11

Delight thyself also in the Lord; and he shall give thee the desires of thine heart.

Psalm 37:4

Confession: Psalm 91

I don't know of a more effective confession in the Bible than Psalm 91. We confess this on a daily basis. The keys to making Psalm 91 work for you are found in verses 1 and 2. You must be dwelling in the secret place of the Most High, abiding in the shadow of the Almighty. How do you do that? Verse 2 tells you: You must "Say of the Lord."

We pray it like this:

Father, we thank You that we (our family, our ministry) dwell in the secret place of the Most High, and we abide under the shadow of the Almighty. For we boldly say, decree, and declare that the Lord, El Shaddai, the God Who is more than enough, Jehovah Jireh, Jehovah Rapha, Jehovah Tsidkenu, Jehovah Shalom, Jehovah Nissi, Jehovah Rapha, Jehovah Shammah, the possessor of heaven and earth, is our God. We trust in Him—some trust in horses, some in chariots, but we trust in the name of the Lord our God. He is our refuge and our fortress, our God, in Him do we trust. Surely He shall deliver us from the snare of the fowler and from the noisome pestilence. He shall cover us with His feathers, and under His wings shall we trust; His truth shall be our shield and buckler. We shall not be afraid for the terror by night, nor for the arrow that flieth by day, nor for the pestilence that walketh in darkness, nor for the destruction that wasteth at noonday. A thousand shall fall at our side and ten thousand at our right hand, but it shall not come nigh us. Only with our eyes shall we behold and see the reward of the wicked.

Because we have made the Lord which is our refuge, even the Most High, our habitation, there shall no evil befall us, neither shall any plague come nigh our dwelling. For He shall give His angels charge over us, to keep us in all our ways. They shall bear us up in their hands lest we dash our foot against a stone. We shall tread upon the lion and the adder; the young lion and the dragon shall we trample underfoot.

We have set our love upon Him; therefore, He will deliver us. He will set us on high, because we have known His name. We shall call upon Him, and He will answer us. He will be with us in trouble; He will deliver us and honor us. With long life will He satisfy us and show us His salvation. Salvation is of the Lord. In Jesus' name. (Ps. 91:1-16; Ps. 20:7.)

Confession: Psalm 103

Father, according to Psalm 103, I say, "Bless the Lord, O my soul: and all that is within me, bless his holy name. Bless the Lord, O my soul, and forget not all his benefits." I say it and decree it over our family and our ministry and all that our family has anything to do with. I declare that those benefits belong to us. We'll not forget the benefits of the Lord: that our iniquities are forgiven, every sin is under the blood of Jesus. Father, Your Word says that if we confess our sins, You are faithful and just to forgive us our sins and to cleanse us from all unrighteousness. So we put every thought, every deed that's wrong, that is not pleasing to You, under the blood of Jesus. We ask for forgiveness, Lord. And we say that we are cleansed and forgiven in Jesus' name. Father, we thank You for that.

We say that You redeem our lives from destruction. We are protected by You, by Your Word, by Your angels. We'll not die prematurely; we'll not be destroyed. The destroyer, the accuser of the brethren, has been cast down. We're redeemed from destruction. Our lives will not be destroyed.

You heal all our diseases. You crown us with lovingkindness and tender mercies. You satisfy our mouth with good things. I say that we have good things to speak and good things to eat so that our youth is renewed like the eagle's. We'll not be old, decrepit, and senile; even though we gain in age, we'll not go downhill. We wait on the Lord, and our youth is renewed.

Bless the Lord, O my soul, and all that is within me, bless His holy name. We thank You for all those benefits, and we'll be careful not to forget them. We give You glory and honor and thanks, in Jesus' name. (Ps. 103:1-5; 1 John 1:9.)

Before Pregnancy:

Desire To Conceive, Fulfillment Over Barrenness

Father, we thank You that children are the heritage of the Lord, and the fruit of the womb is His reward. Children are Your idea, Father; You thought up children, and family, and home. You instituted the family in the Garden of Eden. You ordered children; You commanded them when You said to Adam and Eve, "Be fruitful and multiply." You said that the barren womb is never satisfied. Lord, the Word declares that I am wonderfully and fearfully made by You; therefore, I'm perfect and able to conceive and have children. You said that I/my wife would be a fruitful vine by the side of our house and our children like olive plants around our table. We are not ashamed but happy because our quiver is full of children (or arrows, as You call them).

Thank You, Father, that You designed and fashioned me/her, to have children, that in the Bible barrenness was the exception, not the rule, not Your will, not normal, something against Your plan and purpose. And in Your goodness and faithfulness, every barren woman in the Bible who was godly and believed Your Word became pregnant; You opened her womb and blessed her, and she gave birth to a precious baby just as I/she will. You make the barren woman to keep house and to be a joyful mother of children.

You said, Father, that because You are our God and we are Your people and have a covenant with You, that You will love us and bless us and multiply us and bless the fruit of my/her womb and that neither male nor female among Your people would be barren.

Father, we are redeemed from the curse of the Law by Jesus, and being barren is under the curse of the Law; therefore, we will receive from Your grace and have children.

Father, no plague, no evil shall come nigh our dwelling. We are healed by the stripes of Jesus. Sickness of any kind is taken out of our midst. You said to ask anything of You in Jesus' name and it would be done; and that if two of us on earth agree as touching anything it would be done. So we pray and we agree with You and Your Word, Father, that we will conceive and bring forth a healthy, precious baby to Your glory and honor. We pray all this according to Your Word and will. You said, This is the confidence that we have in You, that if we ask anything according to Your will, You hear us; and if You hear us, we know we have the petition we desire of You. We have it now. Thank You, Father, in Jesus' name. (Ps. 127:3; Gen. 1:28; Ps. 139:14; Ps. 128:3; Ps. 127:4,5; Ps. 113:9; Gal. 3:13; Ps. 91; 1 Peter 2:24; Ex. 23:25; John 16:23; Matt. 18:19; 1 John 5:14,15.)

Now, talk to your body:

Bodies, we speak to you in Jesus' name: You will come in line and agreement with the Word of God. You will respond to His holy Word. You will function properly and perfectly, the way God intended you to. Every part, every organ of our reproductive system conforms to the Word and plan of God as we come together in pure, marital love. Body, conceive! Be pregnant. Cooperate with God's plan: perfect ovulation, release of perfect eggs from the ovaries, through the fallopian tubes, penetrated and impregnated, fertilized by healthy sperm. Good solid attachment to uterine wall and nourished and protected for nine months (40 weeks) unharmed and unhindered. Grow to a perfect baby—spirit, soul and body. Your Word says, Father, that none shall cast their young, nor be barren among Your people and the number of our days You will fulfill. This pregnancy will be fulfilled. We decree it in Jesus' name and receive God's best; we won't settle for anything less in Jesus' holy name. Thank You, Lord, that it is so and done to Your honor and glory. Amen. (Ex. 23:26.)

Now at this point—before conception—is the proper time to build your faith. Don't wait; do it now. Get these Scriptures and truths in your spirit until they are real to you, until you are thinking them and talking them and believing them.

If you want a particular sex in this baby, now is the time to believe for that—not after conception.

If you want a boy or if you want a girl, set your faith early—set it now. Ask God for the desire of your heart.

If you know of a problem in your body, a deficiency or malfunction, now is the time to believe for your healing. Get ready physically to get pregnant.

Speak to your body every day to conceive, carry, and deliver your baby. Do it in faith; don't do it in fear.

These "barren" women "conceived and bare" children. You set your faith to conceive and bare also, in Jesus' name.

Sarah

But Sarai was barren; she had no child....

And he said, I will certainly return unto thee according to the time of life; and, lo, Sarah thy wife shall have a son. And Sarah heard it in the tent door, which was behind him.

Now Abraham and Sarah were old and well stricken in age; and it ceased to be with Sarah after the manner of women....

And the Lord visited Sarah as he had said, and the Lord did unto Sarah as he had spoken.

For Sarah conceived, and bare Abraham a son in his old age, at the set time of which God had spoken to him.

Genesis 11:30; 18:10,11; 21:1,2

Rebekah

And Isaac entreated the Lord for his wife, because she was barren: and the Lord was entreated of him, and Rebekah his wife conceived.

Genesis 25:21

Leah

And when the Lord saw that Leah was hated, he opened her womb: but Rachel was barren.

Genesis 29:31

Rachel

And when Rachel saw that she bare Jacob no children, Rachel envied her sister; and said unto Jacob, Give me children, or else I die...

And God remembered Rachel, and God hearkened to her, and opened her womb.

And she conceived, and bare a son; and said, God hath taken away my reproach.

Genesis 30:1,22,23

Hannah

For this child I prayed; and the Lord hath given me my petition which I asked of him.

1 Samuel 1:27

Manoah's Wife, Samson's Mother

And there was a certain man of Zorah, of the family of the Danites, whose name was Manoah; and his wife was barren, and bare not.

And the angel of the Lord appeared unto the woman, and said unto her, Behold now, thou art barren, and barest not: but thou shalt conceive, and bear a son.

And the woman bare a son, and called his name Samson: and the child grew, and the Lord blessed him.

Judges 13:2,3,24

Ruth

We don't know if Ruth was barren, but she didn't have children with her first husband. She did, however, become the great-grandmother of David.

So Boaz took Ruth, and she was his wife: and when he went in unto her, the Lord gave her conception, and she bare a son.

Ruth 4:13

Shunammite Woman

And he said, What then is to be done for her? And Gehazi answered, Verily she hath no child, and her husband is old.

And he said, Call her. And when he had called her, she stood in the door.

And the woman conceived, and bare a son at that season that Elisha had said unto her, according to the time of life.

2 Kings 4:14,15,17

Elisabeth,
Mother of John the Baptist

And they had no child, because that Elisabeth was barren, and they both were now well stricken in years...

And after those days his wife Elisabeth conceived, and hid herself five months, saying,

Thus hath the Lord dealt with me in the days wherein he looked on me, to take away my reproach among men.

Luke 1:7,24,25

These are good Scriptures for prayers and confessions:

And he will love thee, and bless thee, and multiply thee: he will also bless the fruit of thy womb, and the fruit of thy land, thy corn, and thy wine, and thine oil, the increase of thy kine, and the flocks of thy sheep, in the land which he sware unto thy fathers to give thee.

Thou shalt be blessed above all people: there shall not be male or female barren among you, or among your cattle.

And the Lord will take away from thee all sickness, and will put none of the evil diseases of Egypt, which thou knowest, upon thee; but will lay them upon all them that hate thee.

Deuteronomy 7:13-15

And ye shall serve the Lord your God, and he shall bless thy bread, and thy water; and I will take sickness away from the midst of thee.

There shall nothing cast their young, nor be barren, in thy land: the number of thy days I will fulfill.

Exodus 23:25,26

There shall no evil befall thee, neither shall any plague come nigh thy dwelling.

Psalm 91:10

He maketh the barren woman to keep house, and to be a joyful mother of children. Praise ye the Lord.

Psalm 113:9

Lo, children are an heritage of the Lord: and the fruit of the womb is his reward.

As arrows are in the hand of a mighty man; so are children of the youth.

Happy is the man that hath his quiver full of them: they shall not be ashamed, but they shall speak with the enemies in the gate.

Psalm 127:3-5

Thy wife shall be as a fruitful vine by the sides of thine house: thy children like olive plants round about thy table.

Psalm 128:3

During Pregnancy or Threatening Miscarriage

You don't find "miscarriage" or "abortion" in the Bible. It was not and is not today the will of God for you to lose your baby. God wants you and your baby healthy, whole, and prosperous spiritually, physically, mentally, and financially. God is a good God.

There are multitudes of Scriptures you can pray and confess during this time, but these are good and will get you started. Use these Scriptures and the following prayer/confession all the time you are pregnant.

> And ye shall serve the Lord your God, and he shall bless thy bread, and thy water; and I will take sickness away from the midst of thee.
> There shall nothing cast their young, nor be barren, in thy land: the number of thy days I will fulfil.
>
> Exodus 23:25,26

And he will love thee, and bless thee, and multiply thee: he will also bless the fruit of thy womb, and the fruit of thy land, thy corn, and thy wine, and thine oil, the increase of thy kine, and the flocks of thy sheep, in the land which he sware unto thy fathers to give thee.

Deuteronomy 7:13

Bring ye all the tithes into the storehouse, that there may be meat in mine house, and prove me now herewith, saith the Lord of hosts, if I will not open you the windows of heaven, and pour you out a blessing, that there shall not be room enough to receive it.

And I will rebuke the devourer for your sakes, and he shall not destroy the fruits of your ground; neither shall your vine cast her fruit before the time in the field.

Malachi 3:10,11

Just as I said to you that all barren women in the Bible conceived, I want you to know that every woman in the Bible that conceived gave birth, she had her baby, and she and the baby were healthy. There are two notable exceptions.

In Genesis 35, Rachel, wife of Jacob, had hard labor and died while giving birth. She is the only one in the Bible that it particularly points out a different pattern—hard labor, the exception, not the rule. She had stolen some images of gods from Laban (her father). Her husband, Jacob, not knowing that she had stolen them, made a decree that whoever had stolen them would die. She did.

Bathsheba and David's baby died of sickness seven days after he was born. You can read this in 2 Samuel chapters 11 and 12. David had taken Bathsheba in adultery, and she conceived. David then had her husband killed and took her for his own wife. God sent Nathan the prophet to tell David that he would not die but the baby would.

You do find in the Bible that babies, even in the womb (uterus), were real and alive and known to God. This should answer any and all questions about abortion and "when is the fetus alive."

Luke 1:41 says of John the Baptist,

And it came to pass, that, when Elisabeth heard the salutation of Mary, the babe leaped in her womb; and Elisabeth was filled with the Holy Ghost.

In Genesis 25:23 God told Rebekah of her boys in her womb that,

Two nations are in thy womb, and two manner of people shall be separated from thy bowels; and the one people shall be stronger than the other people; and the elder shall serve the younger.

God didn't just see "fetuses"; He saw men and the nations they would become.

In Judges 13:5-7, God said that Samson was a Nazarite from the womb to the day of his death.

For thou hast possessed my reins: thou hast covered me in my mother's womb.

Psalm 139:13

Thus saith the Lord that made thee, and formed thee from the womb, which will help thee; Fear not, O Jacob, my servant; and thou, Jesurun, whom I have chosen.

Isaiah 44:2

But when it pleased God, who separated me from my mother's womb, and called me by his grace.

Galatians 1:15

Before I formed thee in the belly I knew thee; and before thou camest forth out of the womb I sanctified thee, and I ordained thee a prophet unto the nations.

Jeremiah 1:5

Prayer/Confession

Thank You, Father, for this child. I can say with Hannah, "For this child I prayed and the Lord hath given me my petition which I asked of him."

Thank You, Lord, for a wonderful pregnancy, an enjoyable pregnancy. Thank You that I am in control over my body and the Word has preeminence in my life. I will not be subject to my emotions, but they are subject to Your Word. I'll not have morning sickness. You said You bless my bread and water and take sickness out of my midst. Not only will I enjoy this pregnancy, but my family will, as well. It will be a good time, a pleasant time. I'll rest well and sleep well. You said You give Your beloved sleep. I'll watch what I eat and not gain too much weight. The children of Israel walked forty years in the wilderness and their feet didn't swell; my feet will not swell in Jesus' name. Thank You for what Your Word calls blessings of the breasts and of the womb. (Gen. 49:25.) I'll not have sore or cracked nipples and breasts.

I will feel and be feminine. I radiate life. I glow and am attractive during this pregnancy. My husband and children will enjoy being with me, and I will enjoy being with them. I'll be amorous and loving toward my husband. Your Word says that he is always ravished with my love and my breasts satisfy him at all times. He has no need of spoil during this time and he drinks waters out of his own well, and he rejoices with the wife of his youth, the wife of his covenant—me! We will continue to have a good and blessed sex life during this pregnancy!

This pregnancy will be full duration, full term. I'm a tither, and my vine won't cast its fruit before its time in the field. You said I would not cast my young or miscarry and the number of my days You would fulfill. Thank You that You bless the fruit of my womb. My baby is covered in my womb as David declared. You said numerous times in the Bible that You formed and fashioned our baby in the womb and at the right time You will separate my baby from my womb and carry it gently from my womb.

Father, I declare over this precious one, as I do over all my family, that we are healed by the stripes of Jesus. No sickness, no plague, no evil can come upon us. Your angels have charge over us and keep us in all our ways and lift us up lest we dash our foot against a stone. Just like all the ladies of faith in the Bible, I will give birth to a healthy, whole baby, a child whose heart is toward God and Your promise. And Your command is that if we train this child up in the way he/she should go that he/she won't depart from it when he/she is old. Our baby will honor his/her father and mother and obey; therefore, it will be well (not sick) with our child, and he/she will live long on the earth.

Father, I speak to my body and to my baby—to every part, every organ, every system to function properly and perfectly, fully developed as You intended from the beginning. I declare health, wholeness, soundness, spirit, soul, and body from the top of the head to the bottom of the feet.

Speak to your baby in the womb. It's your baby and is supposed to obey you and God's Word.

Note: At this point, you can be as specific as you want to be. If you know of a problem in your family (heredity, sickness), you can address that. The important thing is that you are agreeing in faith with God and His Word, not just babbling out of fear. The concept of confession is not begging or pleading with God, but thanking and agreeing with Him.

We spoke to many areas, or as many as we could think of:

Eyes: Vision, be perfect. (Moses was 120 years old and his eye wasn't dim.)

Ears: Hear perfectly.

Skin: Complexion, be good.

Teeth: Form perfectly. Be strong, not prone to cavities. (Song of Solomon 4:2; 6:6.)

Bones: Be strong, healthy, straight, none broken. (Ps. 34:20.)

Heart: Be strong, healthy, untroubled. (John 14:1.)

Respiratory system: Be healthy and strong lungs and bronchial passages; no sinus problems, hay fever, bronchitis.

Blood: Be normal, healthy. Maintain the proper blood sugar; no pollution in the blood. (Ezek. 16:6.)

Digestive system: Function normally.

Position of baby and cord: Baby, be head down and in perfect position at birth. Cord, be the perfect length and position, not around the baby's neck.

Temperament: Be full of peace—a calm, sweet spirit and a tender heart. (Isa. 54:13.)

Sleeping habits: Baby, you will sleep at night; you will get plenty of rest and let us rest.

Baby's spirit: You will be tender toward God and the things of God; saved at an early age.

If parents or grandparents have a physical problem, don't confess that on your baby. Don't say, "It will have grandfather's teeth" or an aunt's complexion or any family member's problems. But mirror God's Word to Him. Say to God and to you and to your mate and to your baby what God has already said, what God has already willed and written.

Finish the confession:

We pray for the medical professionals we are involved with that they have the mind of Christ and wisdom of God concerning our family and this baby. The eyes of their understanding be opened that You, Father, lead and guide them how to care for me/my wife by Your Spirit. I say we have favor with them, that they are cooperative with us and what we are doing, that all is well and peaceful and under control in Jesus' name.

Thank You, Father, for this time for our family and time to spend with You. Thank You for fulfilling Your promise in Your Word. In Jesus' name. Amen. (1 Sam. 1:27; Ex. 23:25; Ps. 127:2; Deut. 8:4; Gen. 49:25; Prov. 5:19; Prov. 5:15; Mal. 3:11; Ex. 23:26; Deut. 7:13; Ps. 139:13; Isa. 44:2; Gal. 1:15; Jer. 1:5; Ps. 71:6; Ps. 22:9,10; 1 Peter 2:24; Ps. 91:10-12; Prov. 22:6; Eph. 6:2,3; 3 John 2; Ezek. 16:6; Isa. 54:13; Eph. 1:17,18; Prov. 3:3,4.)

Delivery

Father, as I look forward to delivery of my sweet baby, having enjoyed a blessed pregnancy of full duration, I thank You in advance for Your Word, Your blessings, Your peace, Your presence, and Your divine intervention. I pray and confess that my body and my baby will cooperate with perfect, supernatural delivery, that there will be no problems of any kind. I also believe and declare that my labor and delivery will be quick, short, easy, and painless. I believe and declare that I'll have time to get to the proper place with the proper help.

Baby, in Jesus' name, you move and place yourself in perfect position for birth: head first, not breech and face down. You rotate properly as God intended you to. I command the umbilical cord to be in proper position as well. Body, you function perfectly during this time. I have perfect peace and am relaxed. All fear must go and stay gone for I have God, Who is perfect love and casts out fear. My body will not be tense but relaxed, at peace. I speak specifically to all the parts of my body to come in line with God's Word and will.

Father, I believe that at the proper time for delivery my water will break and my uterus will do its job and begin to contract and push my baby down the birth canal and out into our loving arms and lives. I command my cervix to dilate fully to 10 cm., to be elastic and stretch. To the uterus, vagina, perineum, vulva as well as my cervix, you relax, be elastic and stretch without causing pain or any complications. Accommodate the birth of my baby. Furthermore, I declare in Jesus' name that I will not tear or need an episiotomy. Father, pain is under the curse of the Law, and Your Word says that Jesus bore our pain, so I rebuke all pain and will not tolerate pain. I will have a short, easy, pain free delivery in Jesus' name; therefore, I won't need any anesthetic of any kind. Thank You, Lord, in Jesus' name. Amen. (Ex. 1:19; 1 John 4:16; 1 John 4:18; Matt. 8:17; Deut. 28.)

Baby Dedication

We believe in presenting babies in solemn dedication to God. We see in the Bible that parents brought children to Jesus for His blessing. (Matt. 19:13-15; Mark 10:13-16.) Jesus put His hands on them and blessed them.

Hannah brought baby Samuel to church and presented him to God. (1 Sam. 1:22-28.) And Joseph and Mary brought baby Jesus to church and presented Him to God. (Luke 2:22-24.)

Terry and I, as ministers, have been brought babies by the multitudes of parents and in some nations, we have not only had the job of dedicating the baby through prayer to God but of naming the child as well.

We have prayed over and dedicated our four children in formal church services with congregations as witnesses and also privately both before conception and while the baby was in the womb.

Realize that "Baby Dedication" is your presentation of your child to God forever: that God be first and foremost in the child's life; that God use your child for His will; that God protect and provide for your child spirit, soul, and body; that you understand that your child is God's and is only on loan to you, that you cannot just do as you please with your child but you have commandments and instructions in the Bible on how to rear and treat your child.

God said of Abraham, "I know him. He will command his children in the ways of God." (Gen. 18:19.)

Remember, just because you give your baby back to God, He still expects and commands you to raise him and care for him on earth.

Here is a prayer you can adapt or pray as it is both privately, just you and God, or before a minister in church.

Father, in Jesus' holy name, we come before You on this special day to present to You, to consecrate to You, to dedicate to You, to give back to You, this, our sweet baby that You have given us. Lord, we realize that we are only stewards of this special gift from You. Only You create life. This baby is Your baby. You said I must teach my children of You and Your commandments. You promised that if we would train up our child in the way he should go he would not depart from it when he is old. You promised that if children would honor their parents it would be well with them (not sick but well) and they would live long on the earth. You said they would be disciples of the Lord, taught and obedient to the Lord and great would be their peace and undisturbed composure. Thank You for these promises and commandments. Thank You for our baby.

This day, before You and the host of heaven and all other witnesses, we come to present to You in solemn dedication our baby. We consecrate as parents to not provoke him to wrath, but to bring him up in the nurture and admonition of the Lord. We commit to You to train him up in Your ways and he won't depart from them. We promise to teach him of You, Your ways, Your Word, Your will. We promise to train him by example and demonstration as well as our words. We promise to discipline him according to Your Word. We promise to love and care for him and bathe him in prayer from this day forward. We commit this baby into Your care. You can be omnipresent; I can't always be there, but You can. Your angels have charge over him to keep him in all his ways and lift him up lest he dash his foot against a stone. We pray that this child be healthy, whole, complete, blessed and prosperous spirit, soul and body. We bind the forces of hell and the devil in Jesus' name to stay away from our family in every area of our lives. We decree that Jesus be enthroned above all else in our family at all times in Jesus' name. Amen. (Deut. 6:6,7; Prov. 22:6; Eph. 6:1-3; Isa. 54:13; Eph. 6:4; Prov. 22:15; Prov. 29:15; Ps. 91.)

Testimonies

We've included a few testimonies we've received as a result of the tape we've had out called "Supernatural Childbirth."[1] Rejoice, as we have, with these people; be encouraged by their testimonies, and know for a certainty that what God has done for others He will do for you. God is no respecter of persons. Abide in the Word of God and let His Word abide in you and you can ask what you will and it will be done for you. (Acts 10:34, John 15:7.)

Dear Jackie...

Soon after Jerry and I decided to start a family, we were excited to know that we were expecting a baby. We were very disappointed when I miscarried a few weeks later. Over the course of the next two years I had three more miscarriages—none of the pregnancies lasted longer than six to eight weeks.

As this seemingly hopeless pattern developed, we realized that we had a real problem. Jerry and I both went through a series of tests, saw several doctors and tried medications to determine if something could be corrected physically. Nothing we did gave us any answer to why this was happening.

We knew if we were going to have children God would have to give them to us, but we didn't know how to effectively stand on the Word for our miracle.

About the time of my fourth miscarriage is when you and Terry learned of our problem and began sharing with us principles in the Word we could use to build our faith so that we could receive from God. Jackie, you shared Scripture with me which gave specific answers that I needed. I quoted these often.

With this new knowledge, the fifth pregnancy was quite different. I carried this one past the critical eight-week period with no problem. I had never felt better than during those months of that pregnancy.

In the sixth month I began showing the familiar signs of miscarriage. Just days earlier, I had seen my doctor during one of my routine visits. He told me if I should deliver from that time on we had a "good chance of saving the baby." Because of my medical history, he was monitoring me very closely. I knew he meant what he said as encouragement, but I refused to settle for less than seeing this pregnancy through to full term. Satan was trying to use the doctor's words, along with my physical symptoms, to make me give up, deliver early and risk losing the baby.

Initially, fear came, but I quickly overcame it with the Word that I had been confessing and living in the previous months. Soon all the symptoms disappeared. Praise God for the knowledge I had gained with your help!

Early in the seventh month, the same doctor sent me for an ultrasound because he thought he heard two heartbeats. That ultrasound revealed I was carrying twins. What a reward this news was after winning the battle we had faced just a few weeks earlier.

Jackie, you had also shared with me how you learned that we do not have to go through pain during childbirth. I wanted all God had for me, so I claimed the promises in the Word pertaining to that too. If God could help me carry this pregnancy, He could take away the pain of delivery. When I did go into labor, it was hard to know when it was actually time to go to the hospital because I had no pain.

On March 6, 1977, I gave birth to beautiful, perfectly healthy twin daughters: Tiffany Danielle, three pounds, thirteen ounces and Andrea Gabrielle, four pounds, fourteen ounces. It was as though God was making up for lost time by giving us twins. We are so thankful to God for giving us our miracle in a way much greater than anything we could have ever imagined.

Melinda Davis
Conroe, Texas

Gordon and I have three children, two I had super-naturally according to the Word of God.

Our first baby was born with a congenital deformity of the lower leg and later had to have an amputation. He now wears an artificial limb. Along with that, the whole birth process of labor was full of complications and fear.

Doctors began to tell us they were not sure if this could happen to us again. I then had two miscarriages. All this increased the fear I had.

Then someone gave me your tape, "Supernatural Childbirth." Even though I had been a Christian all this time, I didn't know it didn't have to be this way. After the second miscarriage, doctors told me I was not to conceive for at least six months. So I took your tape and listened to it every day for the next six months. I was determined to build my faith to the place where I knew I could have a baby.

At the end of that six months, Terry was in New Zealand, so we had him pray and agree with us. Nine months later I held my completely healthy baby, who was born in four hours, without complications.

With our third baby, again I had no trouble conceiving. She was born very quickly—just over an hour, with no pain, stitches or complications.

I knew this was the way God intended for women to have babies. Gordon and I are so thankful to God for His Word.

Julie Brown
New Plymouth, New Zealand

This is a second generation supernatural childbirth testimony. Edith believed the Word of God and reaped the reward by giving birth to Leanna.

My daughter, Leanna, at age fifteen years became pregnant. She was a sophomore in high school and continued attending school (one that used paces—independent study), doing so well she started her junior year work. She was ninety-six pounds and five feet three inches tall when she got pregnant.

Beginning in her third month, she started listening to your tape on supernatural childbirth almost every night. She got out her Bible and looked up all the Scriptures and typed them out. She confessed she would have an easy delivery and that every part of the baby would be perfect and complete. There would be no complications during the pregnancy or afterward.

The last two weeks of May she had contractions but no pain. She was dilated to 4 cm. for a little over one week. At her doctor's appointment, May 30, he decided to put her in the hospital June 2. At 7:30 A.M. on that Saturday she entered the hospital—she still didn't even know she was in labor. Her baby girl, Brittini Jordan Savoie, six pounds five and one-half ounces, was born at 10:36 A.M. The nurses and doctor said she did great! They were surprised how quickly she had the baby, especially because it was her first— she was so young and so small. She had some stitches from the baby being so big, but other than being tired, she was fine.

Leanna, with the help and support of her husband, is a joyful mother and a high school graduate!

The same Word of God that brought our daughter Leanna into the world gave us our precious granddaughter, Brittini.

Edith Reese
New Mexico

In my freshman year at high school, in 1973, I watched a film in a P.E. class on natural childbirth. I was so negatively affected by that film and the awful pain that woman was displaying, that I didn't think I'd ever have a baby of my own. I thought I could not handle the pain and would just as well adopt.

Although I realize it's pretty common for a young girl to feel the way I did, I didn't seem to get rid of that way of thinking, even after I was born again in 1978 or after I was married in 1982.

I tried to convince my husband that adoption was the best. I think he accepted that when we were first married because he wasn't thinking of children at that time—but I knew at the back of his mind he wanted to have our own.

Two years into our marriage I was given your tape, "Supernatural Childbirth." I had never heard that term before or that painless delivery was possible, but I was very interested in knowing more about it. I listened and listened and listened to it. By the latter part of 1984, being confident that God was no respecter of people, your words of faith rang out in my heart and mind. "If we're redeemed from the curse of the law, then we are. If we are, we are!" That phrase of faith-filled words brought deliverance to me. I believed that it was true for me (and for every believer, as well).

I shared my faith—and the tape—with my husband, Art. He agreed that God was able and willing to watch over His Word and perform it in our lives. Pain is under the curse, and I was set free from pain and the fear of it, as well.

I conceived in April 1985 and in my sixth week experienced symptoms of a miscarriage. But I stood on my covenant rights and told my body that it would not drop its fruit before the time (because I was and am a tither). I spoke John 10:10 and let it be my dividing line: God placed this baby in my womb to be filled with His life and His life more abundantly. I continued listening to your tape and practically quoting your words of life together with you as you spoke. The week after all the symptoms said I was going to lose my baby I went to my doctor, and he said my blood count was right on track and that everything was fine.

About eight months later at 2:00 A.M. I went to the hospital with contractions. They felt like a lot of pressure on my vagina and all around by abdomen, but there was no pain. My legs began to shake a bit while I was in labor. When I asked the nurses why, they said, "You're trying to be a wonder-woman and probably need a pain killer. I said, "No, I don't have any pain, but I just can't seem to make my legs stop shaking."

After about twelve hours of a lot of pressure on and off lasting about one to two minutes, every three to four minutes for twelve hours, Ashley was born.

No pain! In fact, I kept pushing even after Ashley was already out because I didn't feel her come out of me.

I have shared this tape with every pregnant woman who wanted it. I even gave one to a co-worker while I was working for an airline in Reservations. She became born again while listening to it. She also had a vaginal birth when her doctor said she was too small (and because she had a Cesarean section with her first child). After receiving your tape about two weeks into her seventh month, she called me crying and said, "My bones are moving. I spoke to my body like Jackie said, and I know God is making the adjustments so that I can have this baby naturally...I mean supernaturally." And she did!

Thank you, Jackie, for being willing to share yourself and your testimony with so many of us who have been mightily blessed.

Kuna Sepulveda
Honolulu, Hawaii

Right after my husband and I were born again and Spirit filled, we heard your testimony about how you were told by doctors that you couldn't have children, but because of believing God and His Word, you now had four healthy children. My husband and I decided to believe God to conceive.

It had been three and one-half years since we lost our first child, just a few short weeks away from my due date. We were told by our doctor that I would probably never carry a child full term. My husband, at that point a sophomore in college playing college football, decided to throw himself into his football career and started taking steroids, which added to the complications of getting pregnant and having a baby.

I hadn't conceived yet in over three and one-half years, even though we hadn't used any birth control; but because of hearing your testimony on how to believe God for a miracle, we now had faith sparked in us. Our pastors prayed for us for healing, and in three months I conceived.

Complications with the pregnancy set in right away, but we knew it was God's will for us to have a baby, so we just kept believing.

We were visiting with you when I was seven months pregnant, and we shared that we were going through natural childbirth classes to prepare for this baby. I will never forget Terry's response, "Why have natural childbirth when you can have supernatural childbirth?" He then went on to share about how to have a supernatural delivery by the Word.

When we went home, I listened over and over again to the tape you gave us of your testimony. I made a prayer confession from the tape to speak the Word to my body and the baby even though we were still getting negative reports about the baby each time we went to the doctor. I can't say that my first delivery was pain free, but it was a miracle!

Contrary to what the doctor expected, I gave birth to a healthy seven-pound and fourteen-ounce baby boy, John Bryan Lowe III.

When I conceived again, my faith was built up; I was ready to trust God for a pain-free delivery. I had trouble with my water breaking with John Bryan, so that was one specific thing that I believed God for the next time. I was expecting this one to be quick.

When the time came, my water broke at home, and I went into labor. We set out for the hospital, which was a twenty-minute drive. Fifteen minutes after we got there, Jeremiah Donald Lowe was born. When we got to the hospital and they examined me, I was so surprised that I was in the last transition of labor. I felt the baby coming, and when I stood up, he crowned. In a few minutes the nurses had me in the bed.

I was lying there so elated by the fact that I wasn't in pain that the doctor had to get my attention and remind me to push. So I pushed two times and Jeremiah was here! The doctors and nurses were so amazed at the ease of my delivery, they all gave me a standing ovation after the delivery. I felt so over-whelmed about being free from pain. I just kept thinking, *Well, of course this is how God would want it to be because it was so wonderful!*

The next baby came two and one-half years later, and the devil really tried to complicate this one. I was in labor without pain, and I knew it was time to go to the hospital. When they examined me, the doctors told us the baby was coming double foot breach. They wanted to do an emergency C-Section right away.

We asked the doctors for a few minutes of privacy to pray. They were exasperated and concerned, but they conceded to leave us alone. We then did what you and Terry taught us to do, we laid hands on my stomach and prayed over the baby. We commanded the baby to move and get in the right position in the name of Jesus. We spoke to my body. We did everything we could think of.

The doctors came back in and re-examined me and insisted on a C-Section. Michael Paul Lowe was born by way of a C-Section, a healthy, normal six-pound and three-ounce beautiful baby boy. The following day the doctor came to my room. He told us that when they made the incision, they found the baby head first. We were informed that had the doctors waited we could have had a natural vaginal delivery, which they assured us was impossible, due to the baby's original footing breach position. We saw that as a real victory!

I truly appreciate you and Terry sharing with us about trusting in God's Word. It is true, and it works in my life!

Debbie Lowe
Warsaw, Indiana

It was a wonderful day when I heard you share your principles for raising a successful family. You represented to me a seasoned woman of God who had pursued His will and ministry but without sacrificing your children's well being.

Dennis and I had been happily married for ten years. We were in a traveling ministry, and I considered us quite fulfilled. We agreed in all areas except one—children. I felt that since we traveled full time it was best not to have any children, while Dennis wanted a family. But he knew my answers would have to come from God. He only prayed that God would change me.

It wasn't that I disliked children, but I had strong convictions about being a good parent. Even though Dennis and I agreed on how children should be raised, that didn't seem to fit into our lifestyle. We felt God wouldn't want me to stay home through long separations from Dennis, nor would He want us to leave our children to be raised by someone else. My solution was simply not to have children.

It seems impossible now to realize how I was limiting God. It never occurred to me that there was another way. It never dawned on me that Jesus is the Way, and He could easily show me how to work it out.

In 1979 we attended the International Convention of Faith Ministries conference in Fort Worth, Texas.

One afternoon at a ladies' meeting, a panel of trustees' wives opened the floor for questions. When a woman asked about children, the entire panel directed the question to you, Jackie.

You spoke as though you knew my thoughts and misgivings. Your practical answers brought me such freedom that I was forever changed. Your words showed me that children did not need to suffer because of our type of ministry and travel. Instead, they could be a vital part of all we did and have the added advantage of world travel.

I spent the next few years observing your whole family, just to see how it worked for you. Anyone who spends time with you, especially enjoys being around your children. As a result of the wisdom you shared, today Dennis and I have a beautiful and well-adjusted daughter who travels with us around the world.

Thank you, Jackie, for pointing me to the Way-maker.

Vikki Burke
Arlington, Texas

I listened to your tape "Supernatural Childbirth" for several years before our daughter Ruthi was conceived. I found the principles you teach to be practical and helpful in all areas of my life, enabling me to prepare for a wonderful pregnancy and delivery. I experienced no morning sickness during my pregnancy and, despite the doctors' warnings of a long, uncomfortable first delivery, I was only in labor for five hours and twenty-five minutes.

My water broke and the doctor induced contractions several hours later. They weren't overbearing, but tiring, so I opted for an epidural. The nurses told me I wasn't dilating very quickly and that I would be there for a while. George and I just smiled, and when they left the room, we prayed. I dilated almost immediately—much to their surprise. Through the main part of my labor I watched a football game and laughed and talked with my family! (My mom said I would have had more than one brother if she had had deliveries like mine!)

Again, the nurses were surprised when I was ready to deliver much sooner than they expected. However, they advised me it could still take time. Within twenty minutes I was holding our baby! My doctor really chuckled when only minutes after Ruthi's birth I said, "If that's all there is to it, I'll have twelve!"

With much prayer and use of the knowledge I gained from you and from my doctor, God blessed us with a wonderful delivery. I have recommended the tape "Supernatural Childbirth" to many women and am thrilled to finally see it in print. I believe women everywhere will be encouraged by the wisdom you share.

Nita McNerlin
Katy, Texas

My heart is filled with joy and excitement as I begin to share with you my personal testimony on supernatural childbirth. The Lord has blessed me with two beautiful sons, Dominic Joseph and

Jonathan Michael; both love the Lord and want all that God has for them.

When I first found out I was pregnant with Dominic in February of 1983, I immediately remembered your tape on supernatural childbirth which had been given to me by a precious sister in the Lord.

The first time I listened to the tape, I knew that I knew that I was to believe God for a supernatural childbirth. My wonderful husband, Dominic Jr., listened to the tape with me and agreed with me for a supernatural childbirth, a God-glorifying delivery and for all of God's promises pertaining to childbirth. It was a blessing to have my husband standing with me on God's Word for a blessed delivery. I had a beautiful pregnancy with Dominic Joseph. I had no morning sickness, no complications whatsoever. I listened to your tape while I put on my makeup, daily, for nine months. When it came time for delivery, I was so full of God's promises for a supernatural, God-glorifying delivery. Your testimony was so encouraging; I just knew God was no respecter of persons, and what God did for you, He would do for me. (Rom. 2:11.)

I had great expectations as I went to the hospital ready to give birth to my first son. I had a beautiful delivery with Dominic—very little pain; I dilated quickly and easily and only had to push twice. After I had given birth to Dominic, I thought, *If I ever get pregnant again, I know now what to expect during labor,* and I knew my next childbirth would be totally pain free.

In September of 1985 I found I was pregnant with my second son, Jonathan; he was due April 7, 1986. I was so excited to experience childbirth for the second time. I began listening to your tape again and thanking God for a supernatural childbirth with no pain. Again I had a great nine months carrying Jonathan— no sickness, perfect health. On Saturday, March 22, I went to breakfast with my husband, son and in-laws. We went to the mall and walked around that afternoon. My husband, my son, and I returned home. That evening I told my husband, "I feel like my muscles are getting ready for labor," I went to bed that evening at 8:00 P.M., which is unusual for me.

At 3:00 A.M. the alarm went off, my husband was going to the prison in Muskegon, Michigan, for prison ministry. As he was in the shower, I felt in my heart my labor was starting. I had no real pain, but just a bloody show. My mind was telling me "But you're two weeks early." My heart was saying, "It's time."

My husband met the men at the church office who were going to the prison and told them I was in labor and he wouldn't be able to go with them. He prayed with the men from the church to have a fruitful time of ministry as they ministered to the men in prison. As Dominic returned home from the church office he said to me, "This better be it because if it isn't, it's going to look like I didn't want to go to the prison." At that time I knew I was going to have a baby that morning. I showered, then called my dear mother over to watch my son. I called our pastor and his wife for prayer, and the church prayed for me as well. There's nothing like a whole church body standing with you! My husband and I arrived at the hospital about 8:45 A.M. Dominic and I had prayed for a specific doctor to deliver my child; he was on call.

As the doctor examined me (he was ready to go off duty at 9:00 A.M.) he said, "I will stay to deliver your baby; it probably won't be until tonight." (I was only dilated to 2 cm.) I had no real consistent contractions, but I knew my body was going to have the baby soon.

When the doctor examined me around 10:00 A.M., I was dilated to 5 cm. Minutes later I had the urge to push, and I told the nurse please to check me again. She said, "There's no way; you were just examined."

I told her, "I know I'm ready." She called a resident to check me, and sure enough I was ready to push. No one could believe how fast I had dilated. I felt this delivery was just like one you described on your tape. I had my second son at 10:20 A.M. with absolutely no pain! God is so good; He loves us so much. My son Jonathan weighed 6 pounds 7 ounces, and he is adorable. I love him very much.

It was such a blessing how the doctor had stayed on for us. The next morning when he came into my room he told me I had done a beautiful job. I was so blessed, filled with joy and happiness. Having a baby is a wonderful experience with the Lord, your husband and those you love around. What a testimony to have a God glorifying delivery. I couldn't believe I had Jonathan two weeks early, but I believe God knew our perfect due date. He was born on Palm Sunday, March 23, 1986.

I can't begin to tell you how many people I have shared supernatural childbirth with. I keep copies of your tape in my briefcase and am constantly giving them out to people. What a wonderful tool for people to listen to, so they can also believe God for a God-glorifying delivery. Thank you, Jackie, for sharing your testimony with us.

Amira Russo
Rochester, Michigan

Christians are amazing. When I first heard the tape of "Supernatural Childbirth" I was so excited, I began to tell all my family and friends expecting them to say, "Praise God, isn't this fabulous!" Instead, they looked at me and my swollen belly, raised their eyebrows, rubbed their noses, and generally gave me one of those "Bless your heart, you've gone off the deep end" looks. I should have been used to it by that time.

My husband, Dony, and I had fought the war over our seed for several years. I'd gone through two miscarriages, two corrective surgeries, several humiliating procedures, and finally a grim prognosis: "If you want children, you had better pursue adoption." Now I must tell you, we didn't have a problem with adoption, but we did have a problem in that God had given us several prophetic words about my giving birth. The first week we were married, God had shown me a vision of our son, Israel.

The real breakthrough had occurred when Dony was in prayer one day, and he cried out in his spirit. "God, Your first commandment to mankind was to be fruitful and multiply. Reba and I are Your covenant children, and we expect to be able to keep all Your commandments. We declare the curse of barrenness is broken!"

Six weeks later, I was pregnant! Immediately the skeptics showed up. "Don't get too excited…remember your history of miscarriage." I admit, I wasn't too spiritual at that point. I just wanted to slug them.

Our friends Richard and Lindsay Roberts had stood in agreement with us about our conception and ability to carry the seed full term. Now, about six months into the pregnancy, Lindsay had mailed me a copy of the cassette "Supernatural Childbirth." Here I was fighting hell to conceive and carry this child, and now Lindsay and Jackie were pressing my faith a step further. I guess that's what friends are for.

To tell you all of the story of how God moved in our conception, pregnancy and delivery would make a War and Peace novel. Our God is an awesome God!

Did I have a pain-free delivery? No, I didn't. Did I have a much better delivery than I would have without "Supernatural Childbirth"? Absolutely. Do I recommend "Supernatural Childbirth" to my friends? You'd better believe it. I thank God it's now available in book form so women can study it again and again and get it deep in their spirit. I strongly suggest one for a wedding gift, so it can be seeded in before the pregnancy.

Don't expect everyone to do cartwheels when you share this revelation with them. If they don't, just smile and think the best of them. I personally think it's best to find one or two people who will stand in agreement with you and share your revelation with others after your delivery. That way, doubt and negative words can be kept at a minimum.

God has blessed us with two miracle children: Destiny, our daughter, and Israel, our son.

At age four, Destiny asked, with tears streaming down her cheeks, if she could help us pray for the sick in our prayer lines. The first woman she prayed with had cancer and had been given six months to live. Three weeks after Destiny prayed, the doctor's report showed no trace of cancer! Israel has known all the books of the Bible since he was two. I've never seen children with such pure faith and such ability to comprehend and retain the Word of God.

If you're in a battle concerning your seed, whether in your body, soul, or spirit, tighten up your combat boots! Get yourself armed with every promise in the Word and rejoice...Children are the heritage of the Lord!

Reba Rambo McGuire
Nashville, Tennessee

Conclusion

People often fight for the right to suffer. The Word says you can do things God's way or you can choose to do them another way. You can be sick, and God will still love you. You can be poor, and God will still love you. You can be barren, and God will still love you. You can live in pain, and God will still love you. But God says there is a better way. Jesus has paid for salvation, healing, prosperity, deliverance, and blessing.

God is so practical. God is so real. He wants you to do what you can do, what you can handle. He wants to bless you. He wants to meet your needs. He wants you to walk in health and prosperity and all the blessings that He has given you through Jesus. He'll do anything to meet you where you are if you put your confidence in Him and His Word. God will always be there to back up His Word.

I want to emphasize: God wants to bless you. Never let the devil condemn you or push you into doing something just because someone else did it. Remember, the issue is to have a healthy mother and a healthy baby. Study the Bible and decide for yourself where you will draw the line. God loves you just the way you are, and wherever you are is where He'll meet you.

If this book has helped you in any way, we'd love to hear from you. Send us your testimony, and if that testimony includes the birth of a precious little baby, we'd love for you to send us pictures. Terry and I are privileged to have the opportunity to share the goodness of God with you. If you need prayer, encouragement or just want to share with someone, please write to us. We will pray for you and be in agreement with you for God's very best.

Prayer of Salvation

God loves you—no matter who you are, no matter what your past. God loves you so much that He gave His one and only begotten Son for you. The Bible tells us that "...whoever believes in him shall not perish but have eternal life" (John 3:16 NIV). Jesus laid down His life and rose again so that we could spend eternity with Him in heaven and experience His absolute best on earth. If you would like to receive Jesus into your life, say the following prayer out loud and mean it from your heart.

Heavenly Father, I come to You admitting that I am a sinner. Right now, I choose to turn away from sin, and I ask You to cleanse me of all unrighteousness. I believe that Your Son, Jesus, died on the cross to take away my sins. I also believe that He rose again from the dead so that I might be forgiven of my sins and made righteous through faith in Him. I call upon the name of Jesus Christ to be the Savior and Lord of my life. Jesus, I choose to follow You and ask that You fill me with the power of the Holy Spirit. I declare that right now I am a child of God. I am free from sin and full of the righteousness of God. I am saved in Jesus' name. Amen.

If you prayed this prayer to receive Jesus Christ as your Savior for the first time, please contact us on the Web at **www.harrisonhouse.com** to receive a free book.

Or you may write to us at:

Harrison House
P.O. Box 35035
Tulsa, Oklahoma 74153

About the Authors

Terry and Jackie Mize represent over 30 years of marriage, ministry, missions, and miracles.

Terry and Jackie have been frequent guests on numerous TV and radio programs over the years including PTL, TBN, 700 Club, Richard Roberts, and others.

Terry's first book, *More Than Conquerors,* and Jackie's first book, *Supernatural Childbirth* were immediate bestsellers and have been translated into many languages in nations around the globe.

Terry is known as the "Pastor's Friend" because of his undying commitment to the local Church and office of Pastor. Jackie has been dubbed "Mother of the World" with so many wonderful testimonies of couples having children due to her ministry.

When not overseas traveling the continents, they are ministering in Churches, Bible Schools, conventions, etc, in the United States.

Terry and Jackie founded the *Jackie Mize International Children's Foundation* in 2000 to help children across the world. Terry and Jackie have a children's home in India as well as an orphanage in Romania.

Outstanding healings and miracles are prominent in their ministry as they teach the integrity of God's Word. They reside with their children and their families, which include 7 beautiful grandbabies, in Tulsa, Oklahoma.

To contact the authors, write:

Jackie Mize
Terry Mize Ministries
P.O. Box 35044
Tulsa, OK 74135

www.terrymizeministries.org

Additional copies of this book are available at fine bookstores everywhere or from
www.harrisonhouse.com.

---

[1] You can order my tape, "Supernatural Childbirth," from me at the address in the back of the book. Cost is $7.00 + $2.00 shipping and handling.

Experience the Miracle of Childbirth!

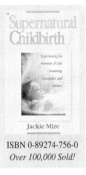

Jackie Mize

ISBN 0-89274-756-0
Over 100,000 Sold!

Whether you're pregnant now or wanting to be, *Supernatural Childbirth* reveals God's promise to you for conception, a positive pregnancy, and a safe delivery for baby and mom. Author and seasoned minister, Jackie Mize had been told she could never have children. However, by unlocking powerful truths and dynamic faith principles she and her husband, Terry, found in the Bible, they now have four miracle children! You'll discover:

How to put faith principles into action for supernatural conception and delivery

How to deal and overcome fear during pregnancy and delivery

Powerful prayers and confessions for conception, pregnancy, and delivery

Inspiring testimonies from women who have experienced supernatural childbirth

And much more!

Available at bookstore everywhere or visit
www.harrisonhouse.com.

Fast. Easy. Convenient.

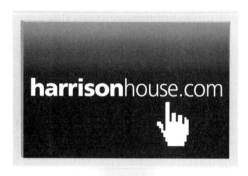

For the latest Harrison House product information and author news, look no further than your computer. All the details on our powerful, life-changing products are just a click away. New releases, E-mail subscriptions, Podcasts, testimonies, monthly specials—find it all in one place. Visit harrisonhouse.com today!

harrisonhouse